The 4 C's

An Examination of Clarity

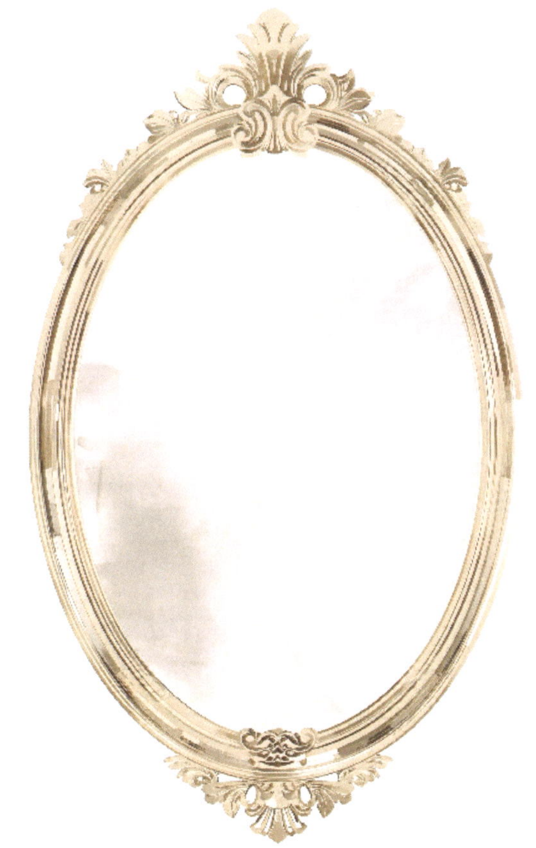

Robin Ingram

Designed by Jennifer Hunt

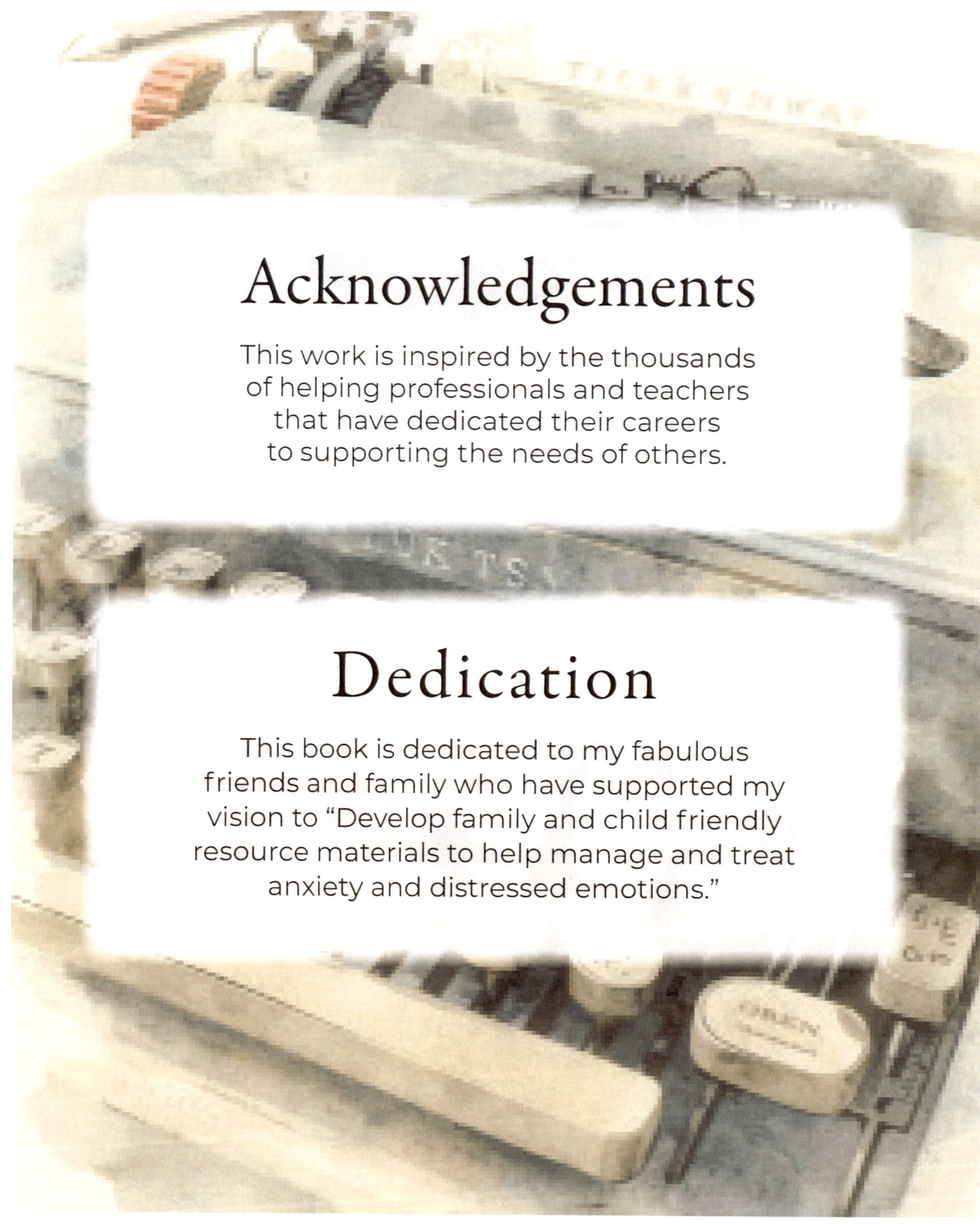

Acknowledgements

This work is inspired by the thousands
of helping professionals and teachers
that have dedicated their careers
to supporting the needs of others.

Dedication

This book is dedicated to my fabulous
friends and family who have supported my
vision to "Develop family and child friendly
resource materials to help manage and treat
anxiety and distressed emotions."

Table of Contents

WHAT are the 4 C's?

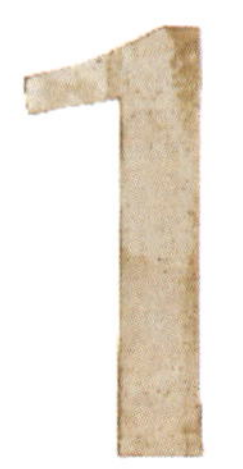

CLARITY
Your wants and needs,
Thoughts and Ideas,
Your Truth.

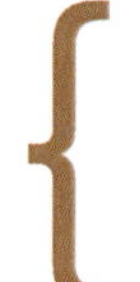

We need BOUNDARIES
to Protect our Clarity.
These are your Do's and Don'ts.

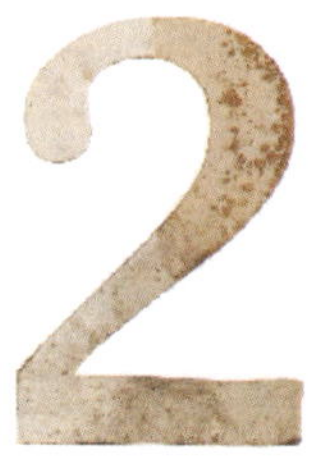

CONFIDENCE
Your belief in yourself
Your ability to follow through.

COMMUNICATION
The way that you share your Clarity
and Boundaries with those that
matter to you.

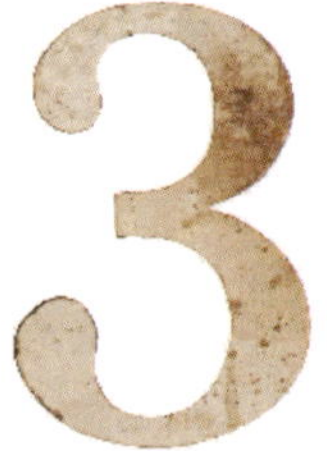

COMMITMENT
A PROMISE to yourself that you will
always stay true to your Clarity and
protect it with your Boundaries.

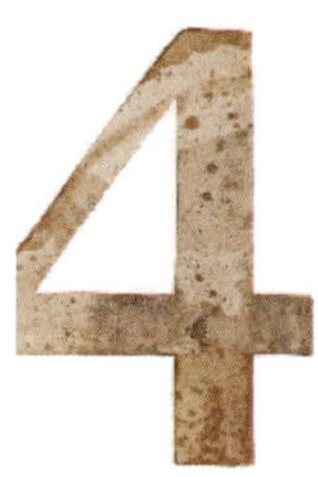

The WHY's

1. With Clarity and Boundaries comes strength and purpose.

2. Without Clarity and Boundaries, we have confusion and chaos. Our friends and family will not understand why we agree to something but do not engage. This most often leads to conflict and resentment.

3. Clarity is our Truth. It is who we are at the CORE. It will most often reveal itself through body language and non-verbal cues.

4. Most of us have not taken the time nor know HOW to Examine our Clarity and Develop Boundaries.

5. This Book will systematically take you through an Examination of Clarity the MOST COMMON areas of your Lives.

6. After completing these exercises, you will be able to express yourself with confidence and purpose, thereby reducing and/or eliminating confusion and conflict in your life.

Let's GO!

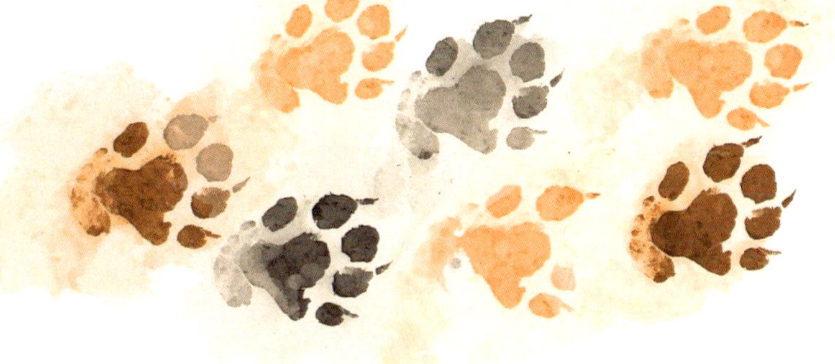

Area of life: Romantic Relationships

Wants and Needs/Clarity

In a Partner, I Want:

____

____

____

In a Partner, I Need:

____

____

____

Do's and Don'ts/Boundaries

My Partner will please me by/The Do's:

____

____

____

My Partner will offend me by/The Don'ts:

____

____

____

Confidence

I will show my Confidence by/through:

____

____

____

Communication

I will share my Clarity and Boundaries by communicating using these following methods:

____

____

____

Commitment

I will stay true to my Clarity by following through and always believing in myself. Examples of my Commitment look like:

____

____

____

____

Extra Notes:

____

____

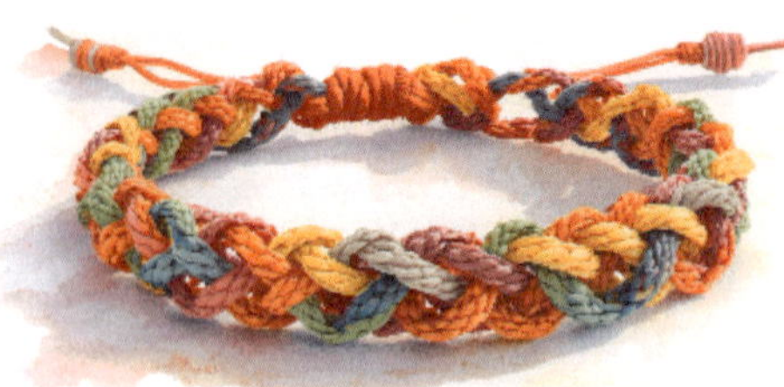

Area of life: Friendships

Wants and Needs/Clarity

In a Friend, I Want:

____

____

____

In a Friend, I Need:

____

____

____

Do's and Don'ts/Boundaries

My Friend will please me by/The Do's:

____

____

____

My Friend will offend me by/The Don'ts:

____

____

____

Confidence

I will show my Confidence by/through:

____

____

____

Communication

I will share my Clarity and Boundaries by communicating using these following methods:

____

____

____

Commitment

I will stay true to my Clarity by following through and always believing in myself. Examples of my Commitment look like:

____

____

____

____

Extra Notes:

____

____

Area of life: Family

Wants and Needs/Clarity

In a Family Member, I Want:

____

____

____

In a Family Member, I Need:

____

____

____

Do's and Don'ts/Boundaries

My Family Members will please me by/The Do's:

____

____

____

My Family Members will offend me by/The Don'ts:

____

____

____

Confidence

I will show my Confidence by/through:

____

____

____

Communication

I will share my Clarity and Boundaries by communicating using these following methods:

____

____

____

Commitment

I will stay true to my Clarity by following through and always believing in myself. Examples of my Commitment look like:

____

____

____

____

Extra Notes:

____

____

Area of life: Parents

Wants and Needs/Clarity

In Parents, I Want:

____

____

____

In Parents, I Need:

____

____

____

Do's and Don'ts/Boundaries

My Parents will please me by/The Do's:

____

____

____

My Parents will offend me by/The Don'ts:

____

____

____

Confidence

I will show my Confidence by/through:

____

____

____

Communication

I will share my Clarity and Boundaries by communicating using these following methods:

____

____

____

Commitment

I will stay true to my Clarity by following through and always believing in myself. Examples of my Commitment look like:

____

____

____

____

Extra Notes:

____

____

Area of life: Career & Co-workers

Wants and Needs/Clarity

In Co-workers, I Want:

____

____

____

In Co-workers, I Need:

____

____

____

Do's and Don'ts/Boundaries

My Co-workers will please me by/The Do's:

____

____

____

My Co-workers will offend me by/The Don'ts:

____

____

____

Confidence

I will show my Confidence by/through:

____

____

____

Communication

I will share my Clarity and Boundaries by communicating using these following methods:

____

____

____

Commitment

I will stay true to my Clarity by following through and always believing in myself. Examples of my Commitment look like:

____

____

____

____

Extra Notes:

____

____

Area of life: Health & Wellness

Wants and Needs/Clarity

For my Health and Wellness, I Want:

____

____

____

For my Health and Wellness, I Need:

____

____

____

Do's and Don'ts/Boundaries

My Friends and Family will please me by/The Do's:

____

____

____

My Friends and Family will offend me by/The Don'ts:

____

____

____

Confidence

I will show my Confidence by/through:

____

____

____

Communication

I will share my Clarity and Boundaries by communicating using these following methods:

____

____

____

Commitment

I will stay true to my Clarity by following through and always believing in myself. Examples of my Commitment look like:

____

____

____

____

Extra Notes:

____

____

Area of life: Parenting

Wants and Needs/Clarity

As a Parent, I Want:

____

____

____

As a Parent, I Need:

____

____

____

Do's and Don'ts/Boundaries

My Friends, Family and Children will support me by/The Do's:

____

____

____

My Friends, Family and Children will offend me by/The Don'ts:

____

____

____

Confidence

I will show my Confidence by/through:

____

____

____

Communication

I will share my Clarity and Boundaries by communicating using these following methods:

____

____

____

Commitment

I will stay true to my Clarity by following through and always believing in myself. Examples of my Commitment look like:

____

____

____

____

Extra Notes:

____

____

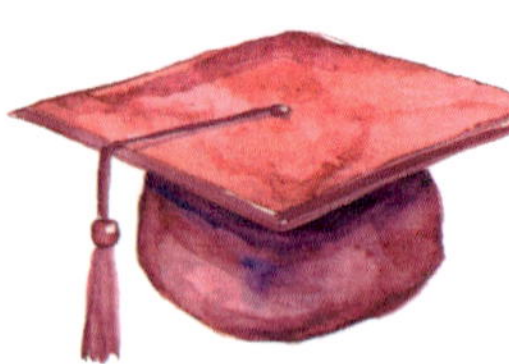

Area of life: Education & Learning

Wants and Needs/Clarity

For my learning, I Want:

____

____

____

For my learning, I Need:

____

____

____

Do's and Don'ts/Boundaries

My Friends, Family and Teachers will support me by/The Do's:

____

____

____

My Friends, Family and Teachers will offend me by/The Don'ts:

____

____

____

Confidence

I will show my Confidence by/through:

____

____

____

Communication

I will share my Clarity and Boundaries by communicating using these following methods:

____

____

____

Commitment

I will stay true to my Clarity by following through and always believing in myself. Examples of my Commitment look like:

____

____

____

____

Extra Notes:

____

____

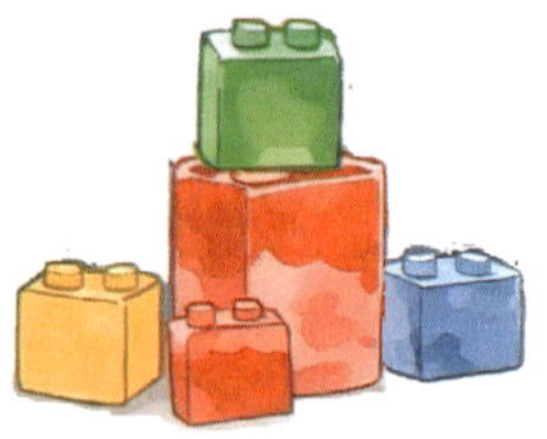

Area of life: Social Development

Wants and Needs/Clarity

Socially, I Want:

____

____

____

Socially, I Need:

____

____

____

Do's and Don'ts/Boundaries

My Friends, Family will support me by/The Do's:

____

____

____

My Friends, Family will offend me by/The Don'ts:

____

____

____

Confidence

I will show my Confidence by/through:

____

____

____

Communication

I will share my Clarity and Boundaries by communicating using these following methods:

____

____

____

Commitment

I will stay true to my Clarity by following through and always believing in myself. Examples of my Commitment look like:

____

____

____

____

Extra Notes:

____

____

Area of life: Recreation

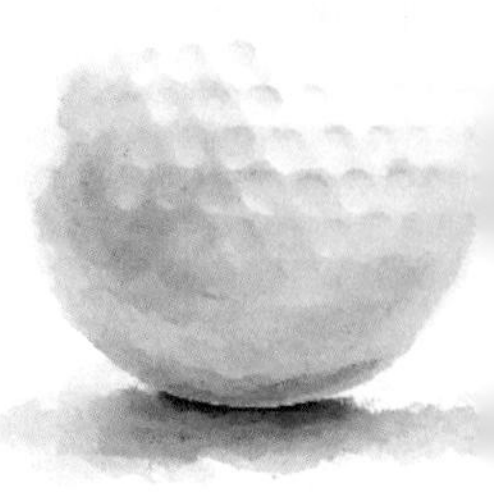

Wants and Needs/Clarity

Recreationally, I Want:

____

____

____

Recreationally, I Need:

____

____

____

Do's and Don'ts/Boundaries

My Friends and Family will support me by/The Do's:

____

____

____

My Friends and Family will offend me by/The Don'ts:

____

____

____

Confidence

I will show my Confidence by/through:

____

____

____

Communication

I will share my Clarity and Boundaries by communicating using these following methods:

____

____

____

Commitment

I will stay true to my Clarity by following through and always believing in myself. Examples of my Commitment look like:

____

____

____

____

Extra Notes:

____

____

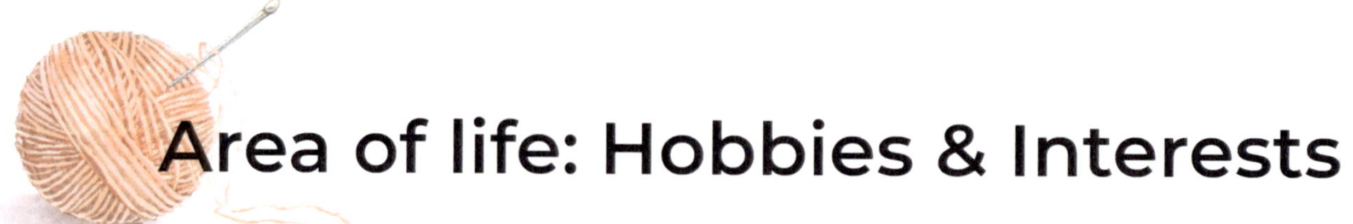

Area of life: Hobbies & Interests

Wants and Needs/Clarity

For Hobbies and Interests, I Want:

____

____

____

For Hobbies and Interests, I Need:

____

____

____

Do's and Don'ts/Boundaries

My Friends and Family will support me by/The Do's:

____

____

____

My Friends and Family will offend me by/The Don'ts:

____

____

____

Confidence

I will show my Confidence by/through:

____

____

____

Communication

I will share my Clarity and Boundaries by communicating using these following
methods:

____

____

____

Commitment

I will stay true to my Clarity by following through and always believing in myself.
Examples of my Commitment look like:

____

____

____

____

Extra Notes:

____

____

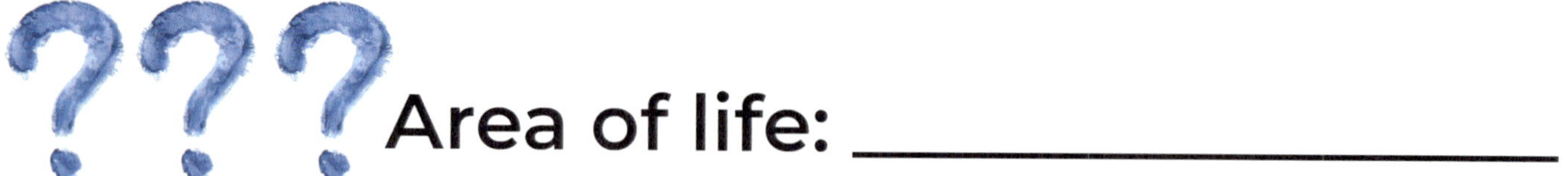 # Area of life: ________________________

Wants and Needs/Clarity

In this Area, I Want:

____

____

____

In this Area, I Need:

____

____

____

Do's and Don'ts/Boundaries

My Friends and Family will support me by/The Do's:

____

____

____

My Friends and Family will offend me by/The Don'ts:

____

____

____

Confidence

I will show my Confidence by/through:

____

____

____

Communication

I will share my Clarity and Boundaries by communicating using these following methods:

____

____

____

Commitment

I will stay true to my Clarity by following through and always believing in myself. Examples of my Commitment look like:

____

____

____

____

Extra Notes:

____

____

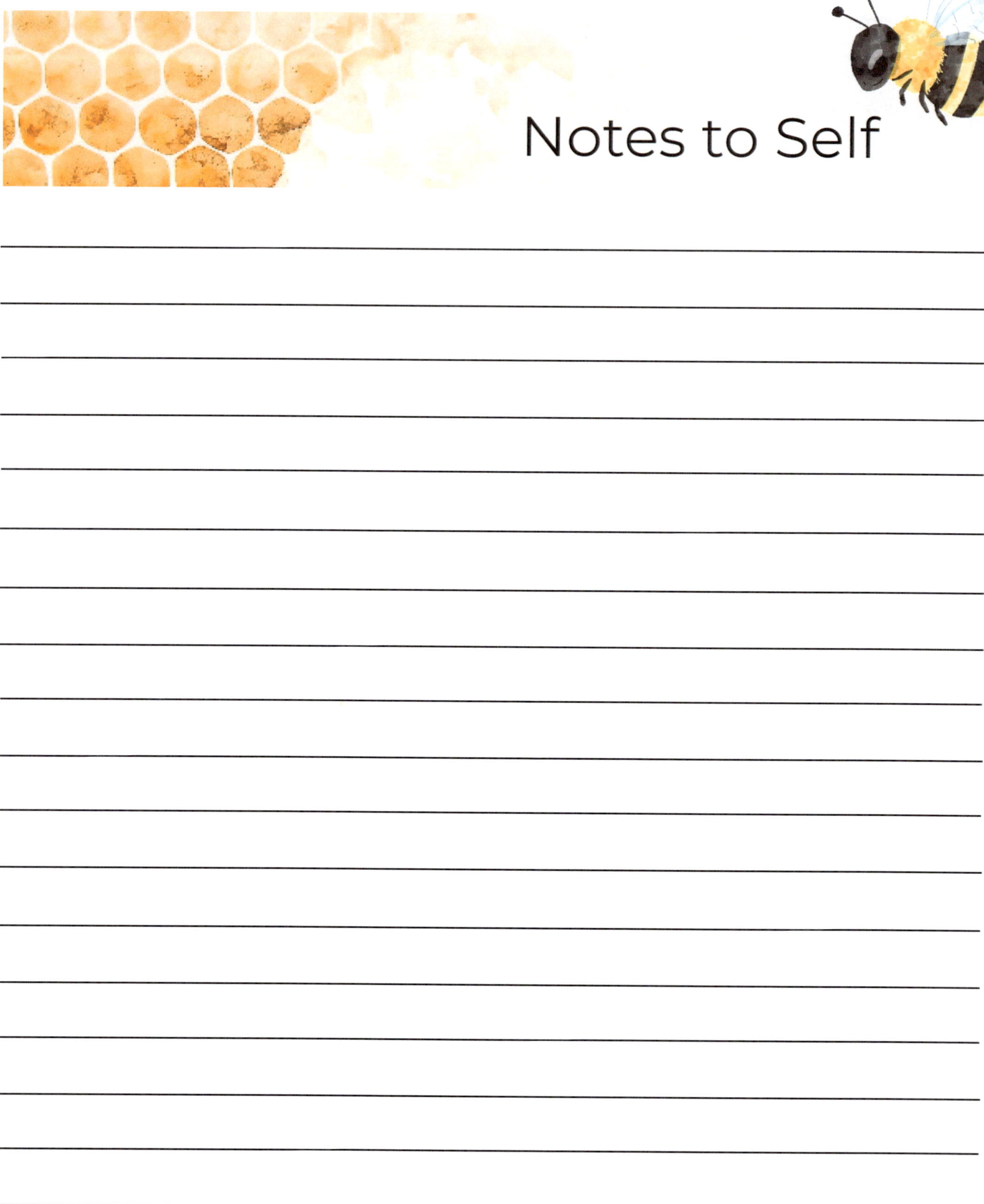

Notes to Self

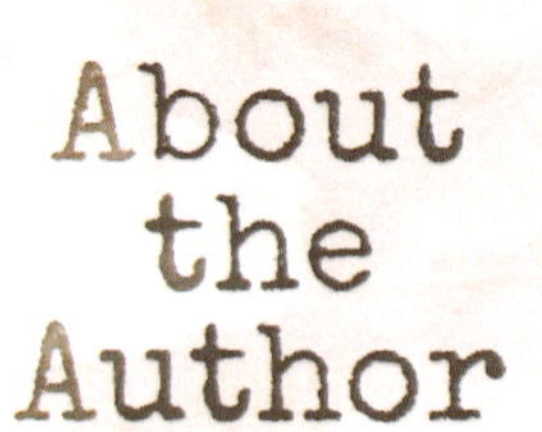

Robin S. Ingram, EdM is the Owner and CEO of a local New Mexico based counseling agency. Her credentials include published author, Licensed Professional Clinical Counselor (LPCC), Licensed School Counselor (Level 3) K-12 and Licensed School Administrator K-12.

Ms. Ingram has a proven record of success as a Licensed Family Counselor, Therapist and Educator with ages 3-103. Her expertise includes Children and Adult Individual and Group Counseling, Social/Emotional Support, Programs Development, Community Collaboration and Outreach, Classroom Presentations, Parent Classes and Professional Workshops.

The areas of specialties include; Behavioral Regulation, ADD, ADHD, OCD, ODD, Anxiety, Depression, Trauma, Eating Disorders, Harm to Self-Behaviors, Grief and Loss, Gifted Challenges, Emotional Dysregulation, Pet Grief Support, Insomnia, Diet and Nutrition, Chronic Pain, Depression, Couples Counseling, Parenting Supports, Social Anxiety, Language Development, Academic Supports, Bi Polar, Education and Career Planning.

Therepeutic Interventions Include; Play Therapy, Equine Therapy, Animal Therapy, Art Therapy, Cognitive Reframing, Communication Skills, Compliance Issues, DBT (Dialetic Behavior Therapy) and CBT (Cognative Behavior Therapy), MST (Multi Systems Therapy), Exploration of Coping Patterns, Exploration of Emotions, Exploration of Relationship Patterns, Mindfulness Training, Preventative Services, Psycho-Education, Role-Play/Behavioral Rehearsal, Interactive Feedback, Preventative Services, Structured Problem Solving, Supportive Reflection and Symptom Management.

Ms. Ingram's Out Reach Supports Include: Workshops, On-site Presentations, On-site visits to Nursing homes, Hospitals and Medical Clinics, Collaboration Meetings, Trainings, Video Classes and Workshops, In-home Visits, and Concierge Options.

Ms. Ingram is delighted to create this much-needed quick-start guide and share her knowledge with all those who seek help.